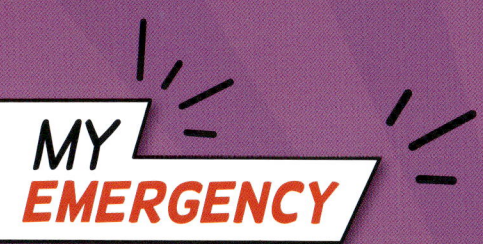

MY EMERGENCY

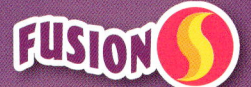

AUTISTIC DISTRESS

By Charis Mather

Consultant: Nikki Forbes, Occupational Therapist

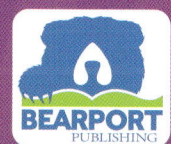

BEARPORT
PUBLISHING

Minneapolis, Minnesota

Photo Credits:
Images are courtesy of Shutterstock.com.
With thanks to Getty Images, Thinkstock Photo, and iStockphoto.

Front cover – michaeljung, ElephantCastle. 4–5 – Photographee.eu, Prostock-studio, Irina Strelnikova. 6–7 – NOTE OMG, STUDIO GRAND WEB, Syda Productions. 8–9 – Photographee.eu, Yuliya Evstratenko. 10–11 – YanLev, Volurol, ArtFamily. 12–13 – Drazen Zigic, LeManna, Vitali Michkou, Ilike, Nataly Mayak, Anne Richard, Photographee.eu, InesBazdar. 14–15 – pathdoc, Alina Tanya, Stockbusters, wavebreakmedia. 16–17 – Golubovy, Dmitry Lobanov, Zapylaiev Kostiantyn, Ekaterina Pokrovsky, TeodorLazarev, Sergey Novikov, Anatoliy Karlyuk, MIA Studio, Veja, 3445128471. 18–19 – YAKOBCHUK VIACHESLAV, Dubova, kornnphoto. 20–21 – Veja, Tatiana Gordievskaia. 22–23 – Liderina, EZ-Stock Studio.

Library of Congress Cataloging-in-Publication Data is available at www.loc.gov or upon request from the publisher.

ISBN: 978-1-63691-969-0 (hardcover)
ISBN: 978-1-63691-974-4 (paperback)
ISBN: 978-1-63691-979-9 (ebook)

© 2023 Booklife Publishing
This edition is published by arrangement with Booklife Publishing.

North American adaptations © 2023 Bearport Publishing Company. All rights reserved. No part of this publication may be reproduced in whole or in part, stored in any retrieval system, or transmitted in any form or by any means, electronic, mechanical, photocopying, recording, or otherwise, without written permission from the publisher.

For more information, write to Bearport Publishing, 5357 Penn Avenue South, Minneapolis, MN 55419. Printed in the United States of America.

CONTENTS

Would You Know What to Do? 4
What Is Autism? 6
What Is an Autistic Meltdown? 10
Triggers 12
Rumbling Stage 14
Meltdown 16
How Can You Help? 18
How We Feel 20
What Next? 22
Living with Autism 23
Glossary 24
Index 24

WOULD YOU KNOW WHAT TO DO?

Have you ever seen an emergency? This is when someone needs help because of something dangerous that is happening.

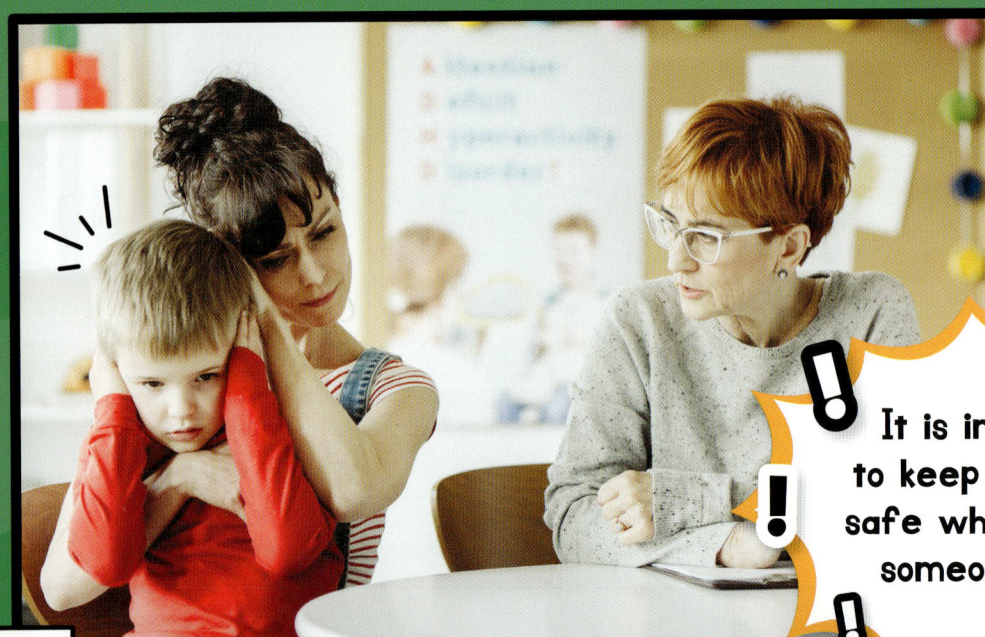

It is important to keep ourselves safe when helping someone else.

People with autism can sometimes have an emergency known as an autistic **meltdown**. Then, they need people to help keep them calm and safe.

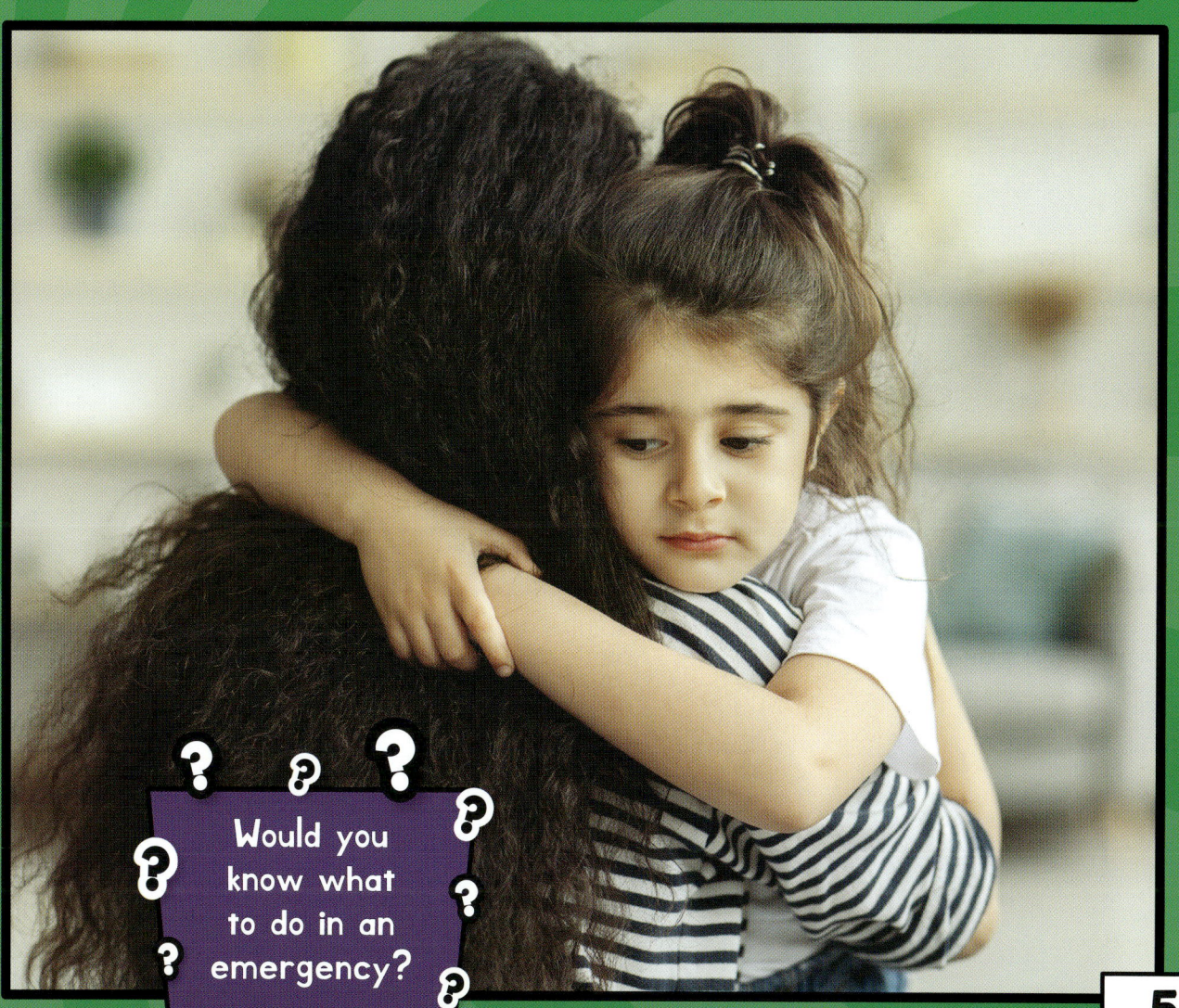

Would you know what to do in an emergency?

WHAT IS AUTISM?

Autism is a difference in someone's brain. It changes how they experience the world. They understand things in a different way than most people.

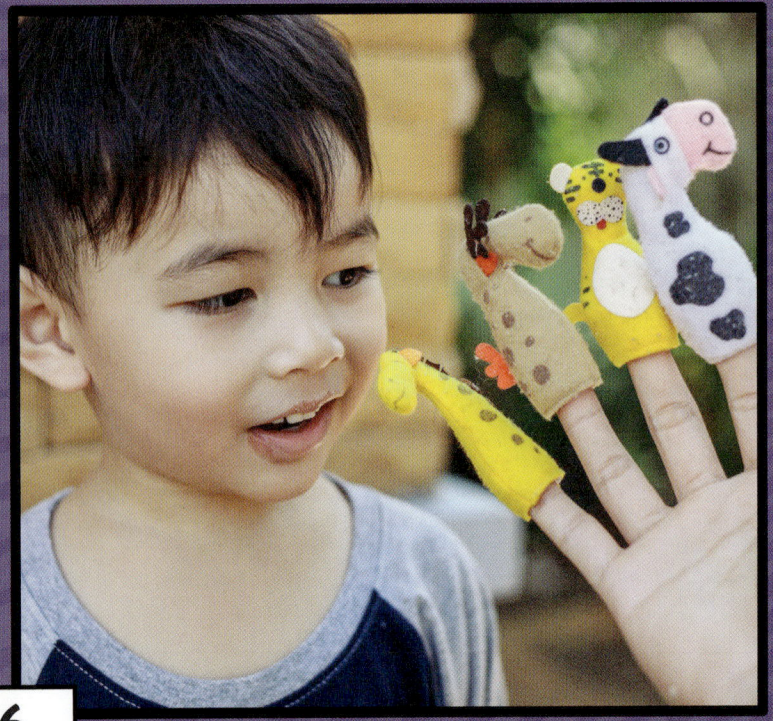
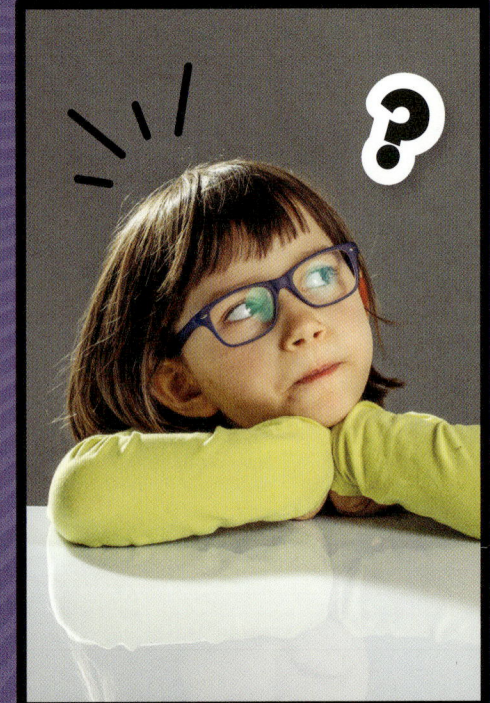

There are many children and adults who have autism. Autism is not the same for everyone. Some people have difficulty being around people. Others have a hard time in places where there is too much happening.

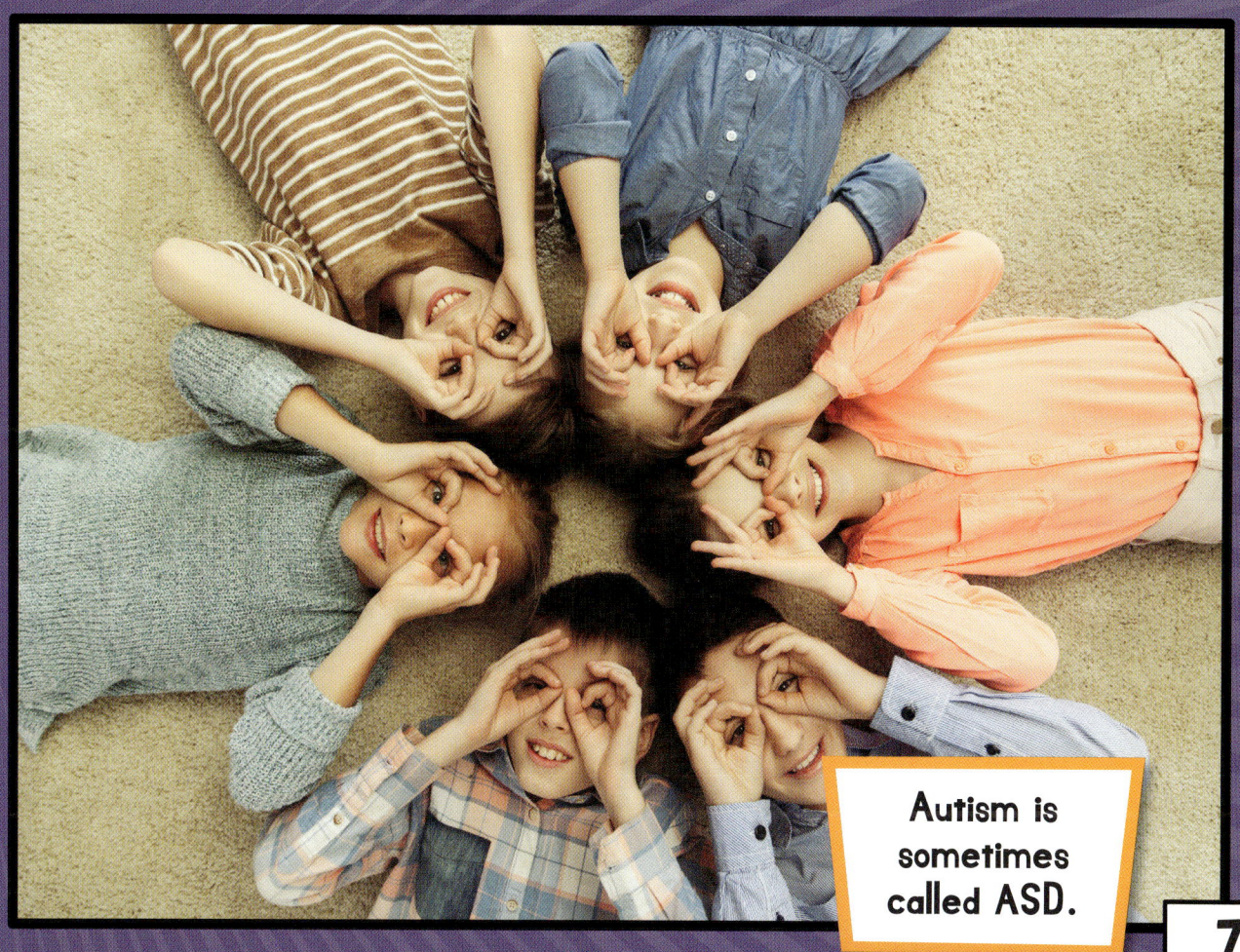

Autism is sometimes called ASD.

Sometimes, it can be hard for some people with autism to **communicate** in the same way as others. They may react to things around them more strongly.

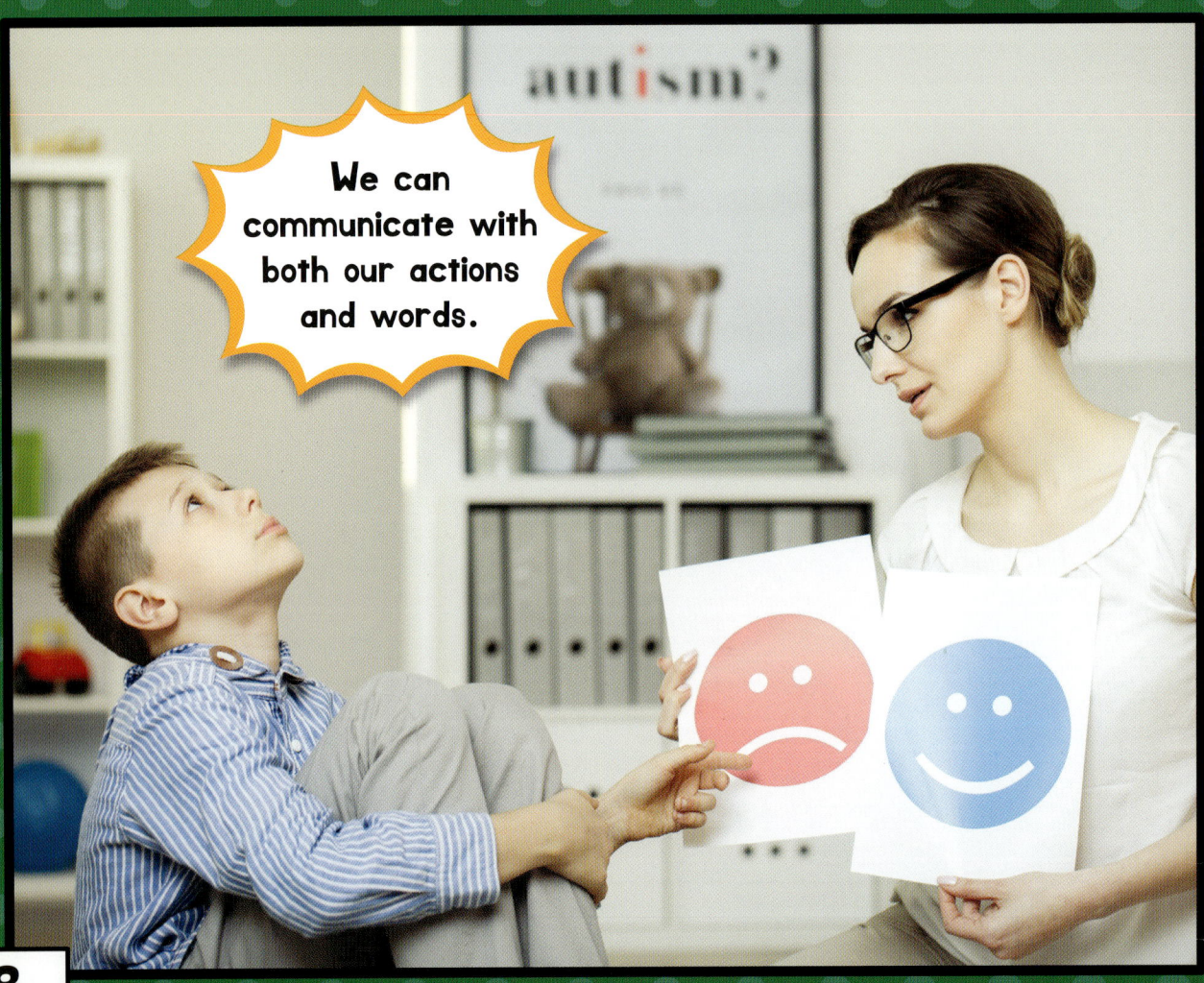

We can communicate with both our actions and words.

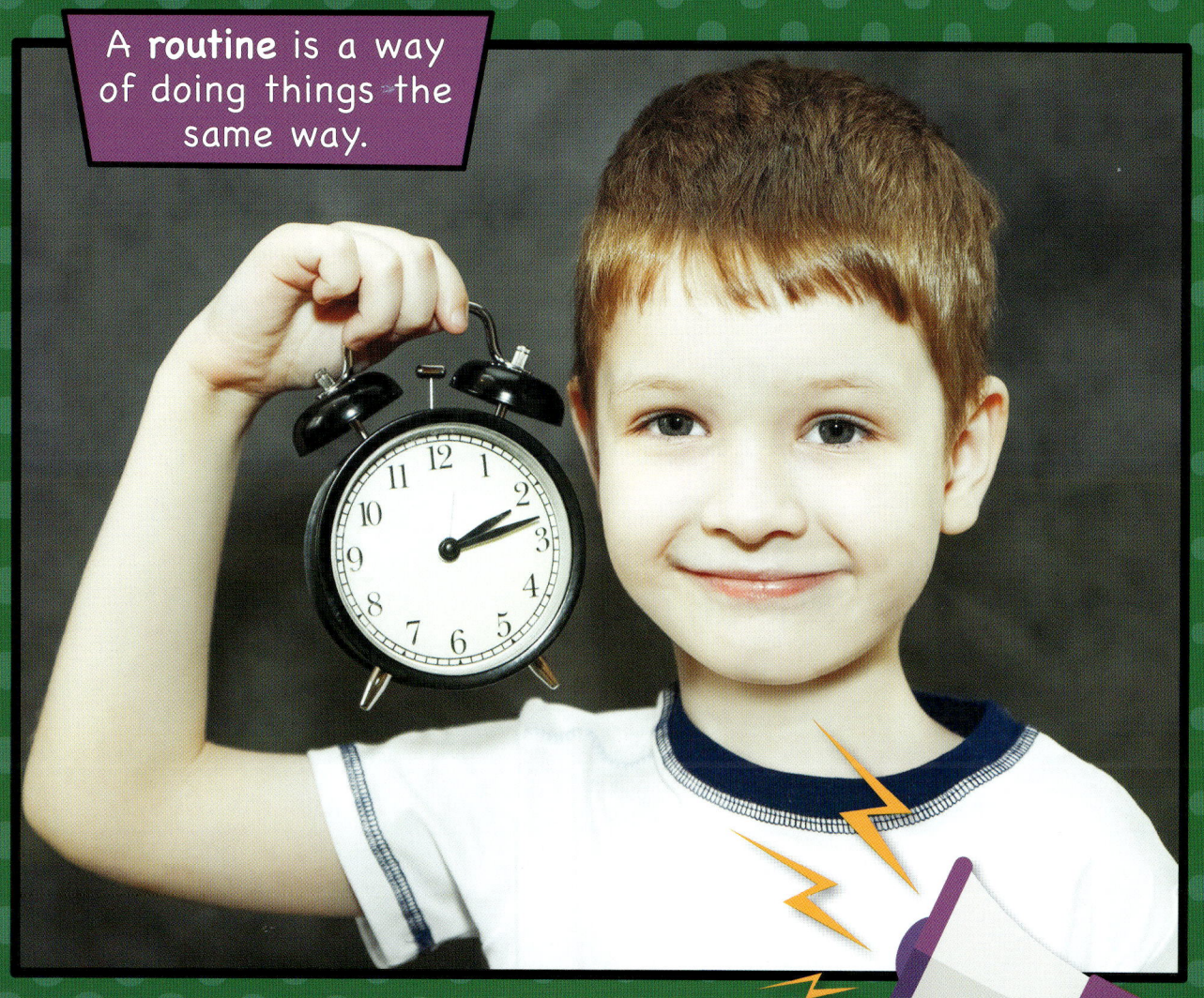

A **routine** is a way of doing things the same way.

Many people with autism find it helpful to have a routine. When things stay the same, it can help them feel calm.

WHAT IS AN AUTISTIC MELTDOWN?

People with autism can sometimes have strong **emotions** they cannot control. This is called a meltdown. Meltdowns happen when someone feels **anxious**.

A meltdown can last for just minutes or for hours.

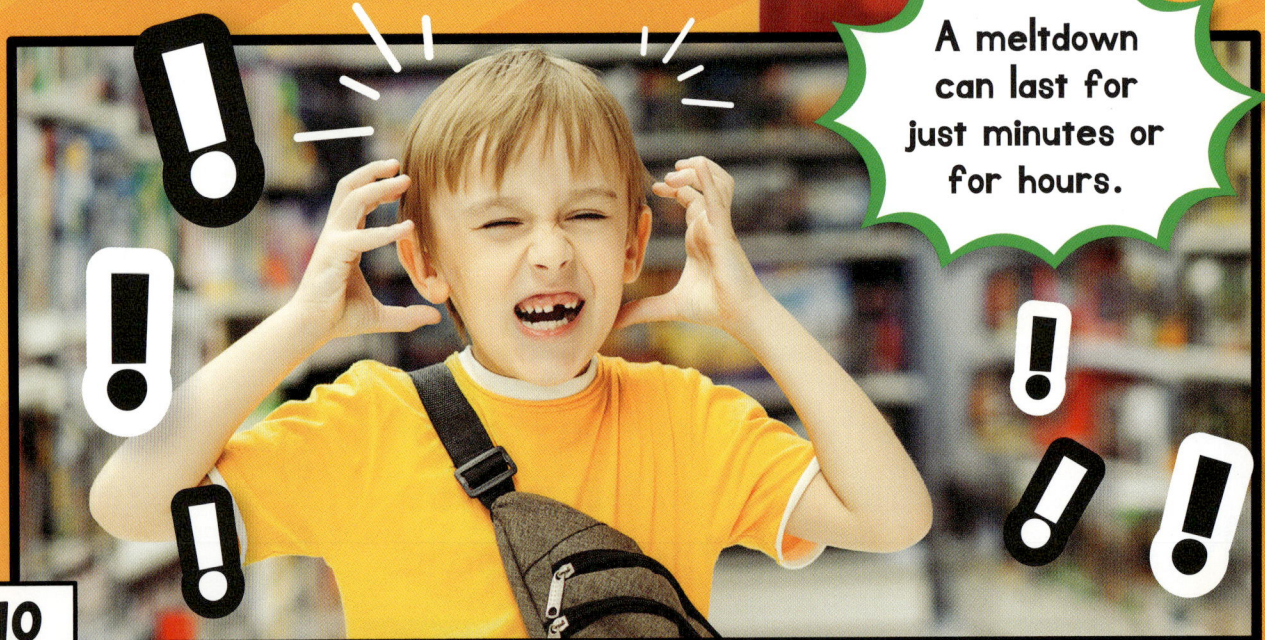

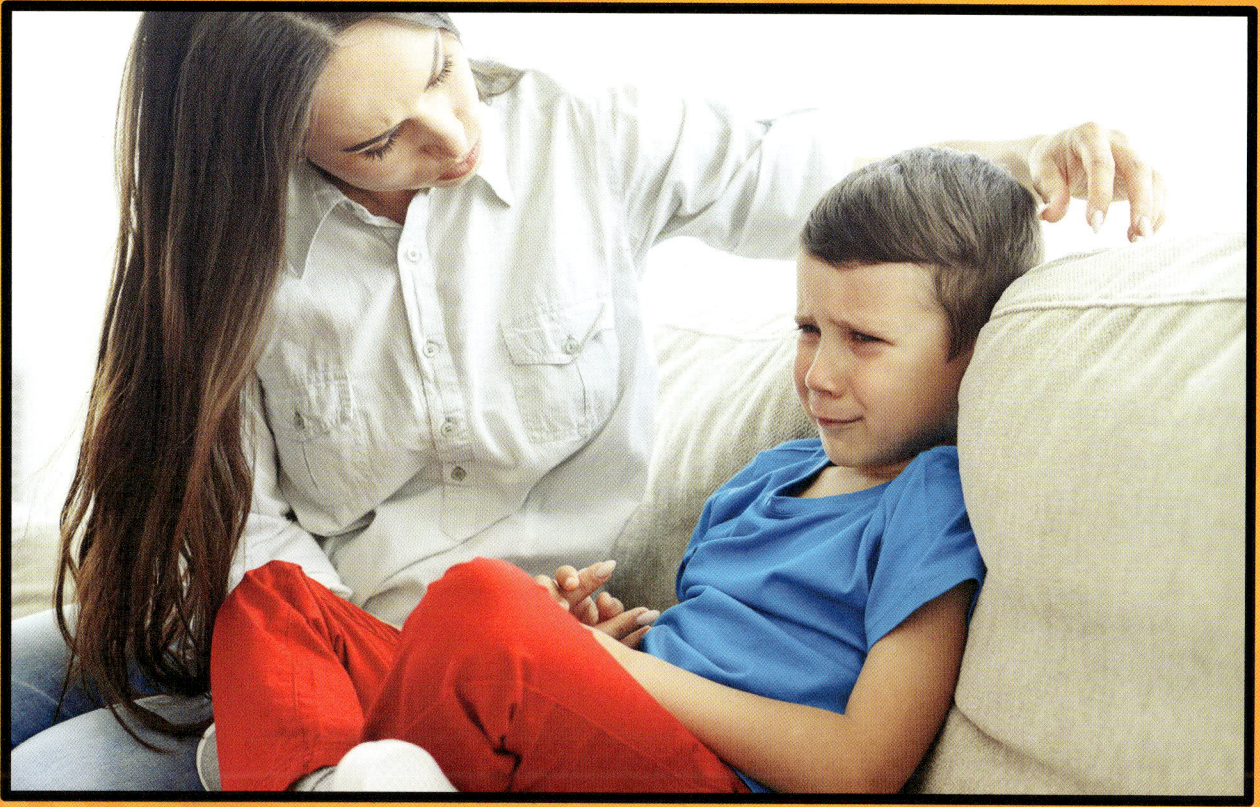

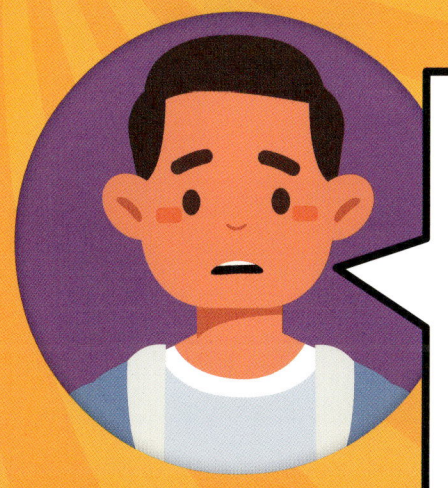

A person with a meltdown is not trying to cause problems or be bad. A meltdown is a sign that someone with autism is **overwhelmed** by emotions. They need help calming down.

TRIGGERS

Something that causes a person with autism to get very upset is called a trigger. Things that seem small to **neurotypical** people can become triggers for people with autism.

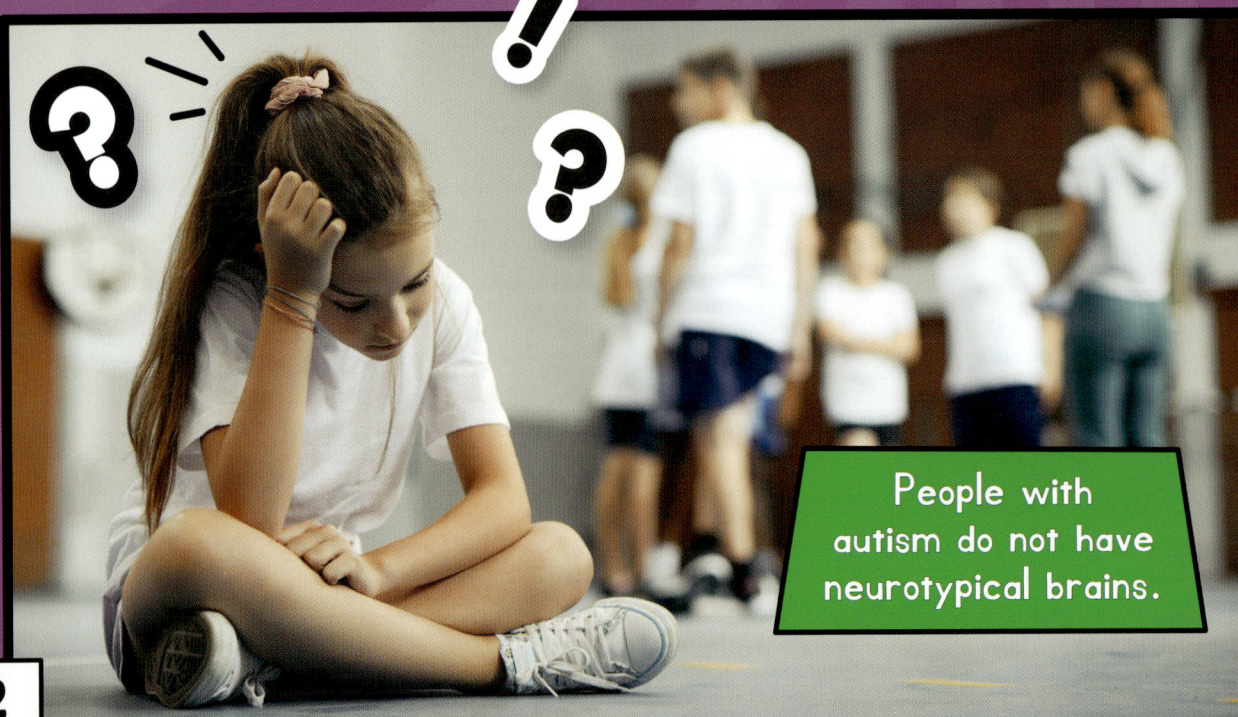

People with autism do not have neurotypical brains.

Everyone is different, but what are some triggers?

STRESSFUL SITUATIONS

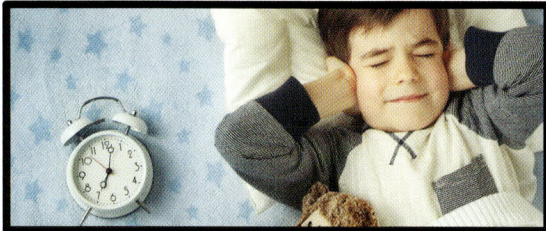
Changes in routine

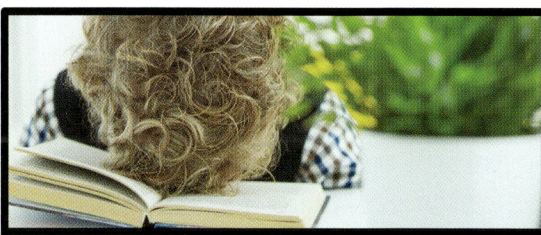
Not understanding something

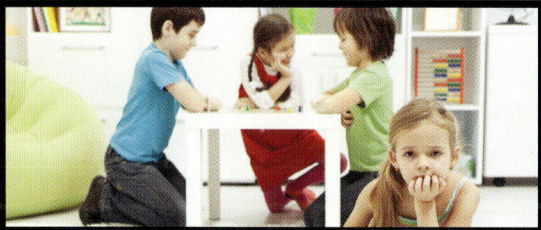
Too many people

TOO MUCH HAPPENING AROUND THEM

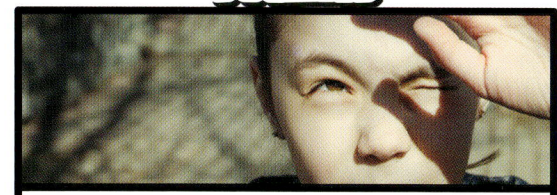
Bright lights

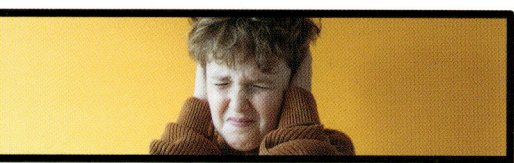
Loud noises

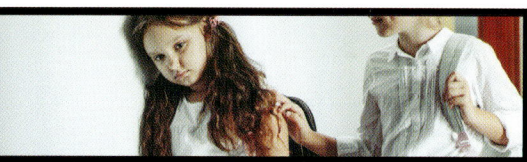
Being touched

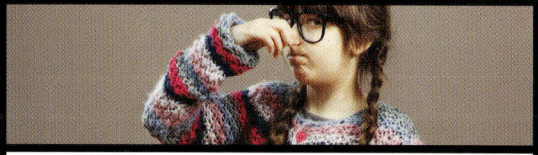
Smells

RUMBLING STAGE

When someone is close to losing control of their emotions, they start to look upset and uncomfortable. This is called the rumbling stage.

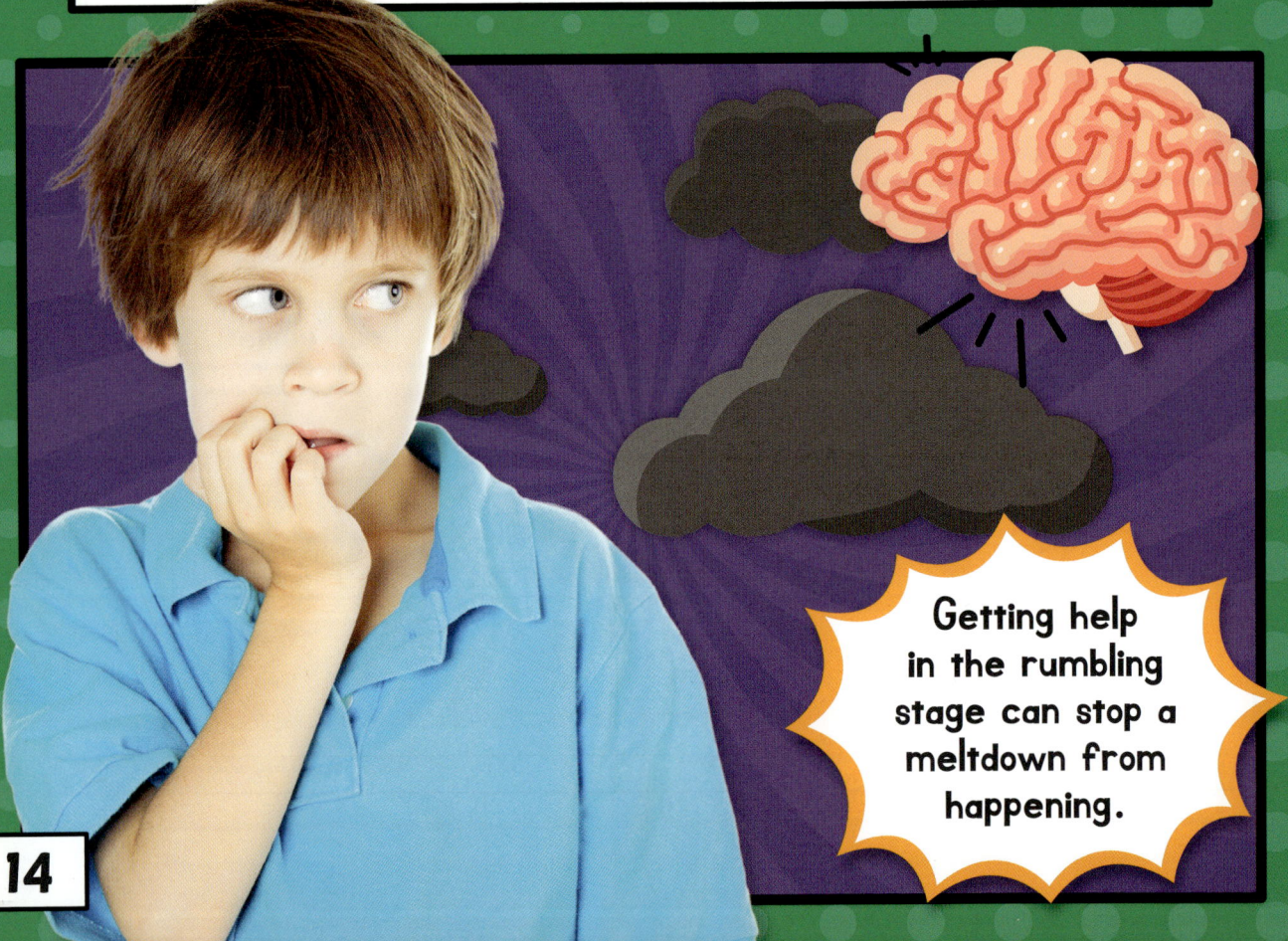

Getting help in the rumbling stage can stop a meltdown from happening.

In the rumbling stage, someone might look very uncomfortable. They might try to be alone or move around a lot.

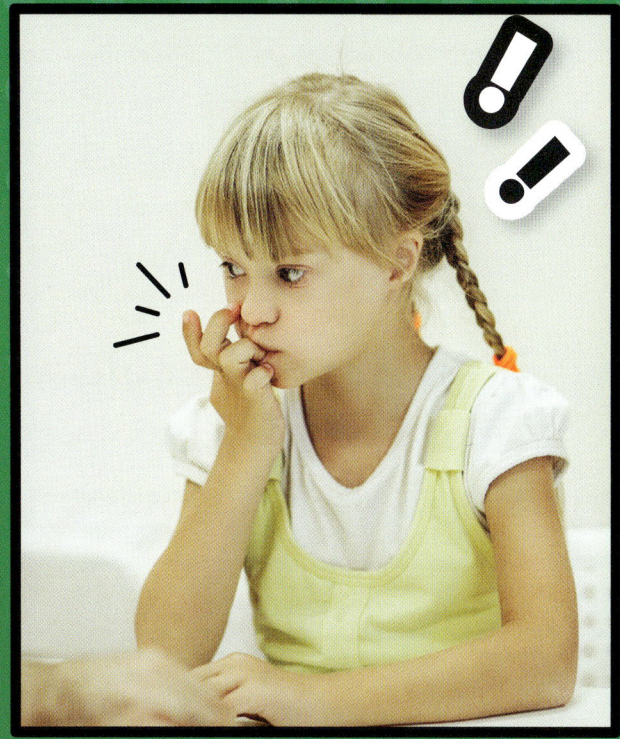

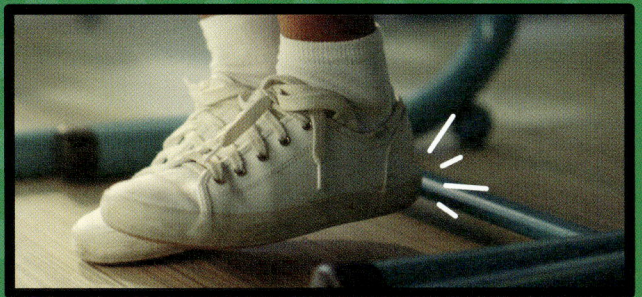

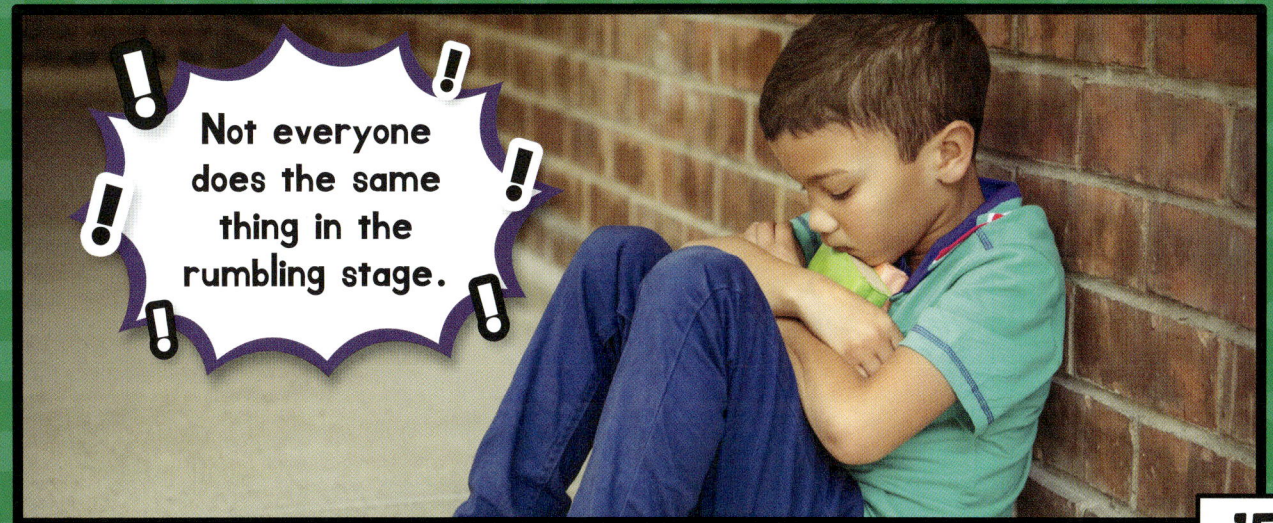

Not everyone does the same thing in the rumbling stage.

MELTDOWN

If someone with autism does not get help while they are in the rumbling stage, they may have a meltdown.

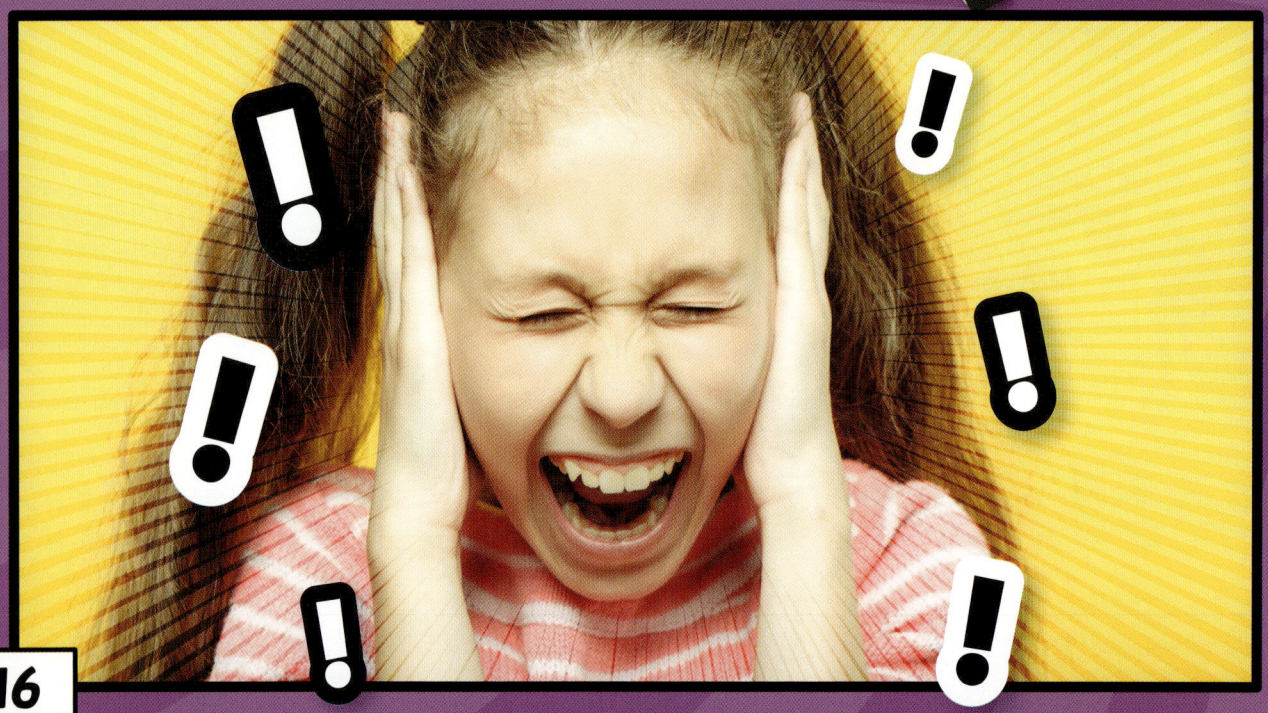

What might someone do during a meltdown?

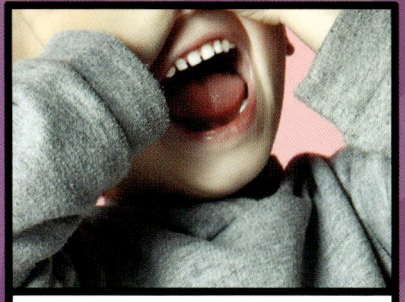 Shout

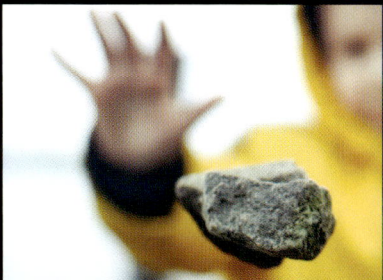 Throw things

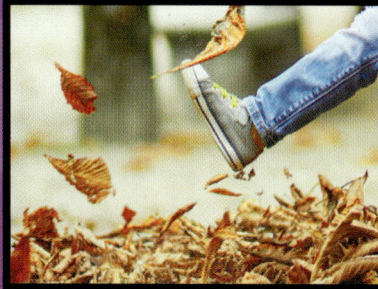 Hit or kick things

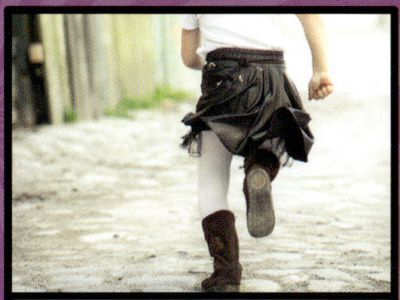 Run

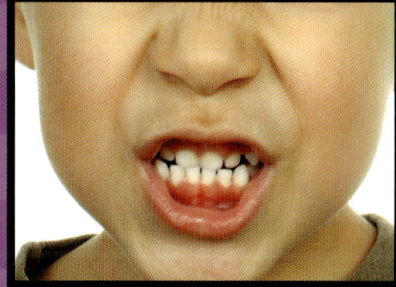 Bite things

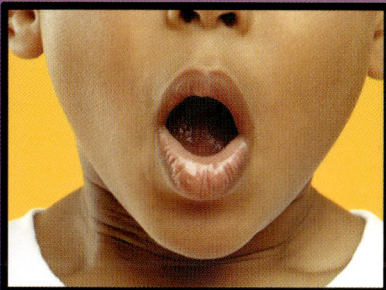 Breathe quickly

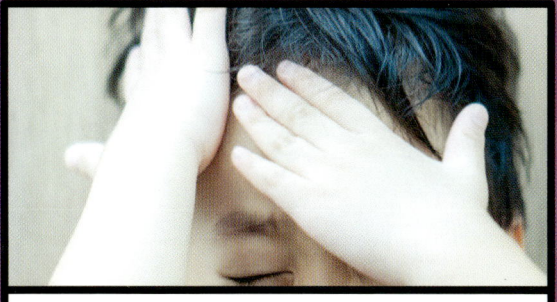 Hit their head

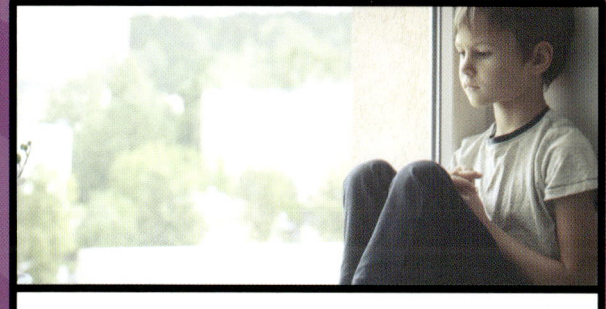 Spend time alone

HOW CAN YOU HELP?

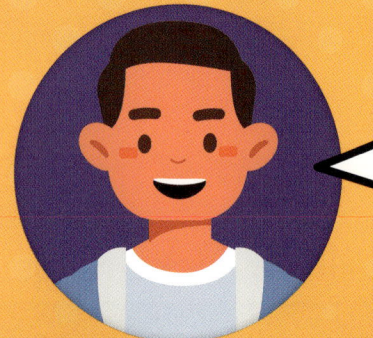

If someone has a meltdown, get a grown-up. An adult can make sure everyone stays safe.

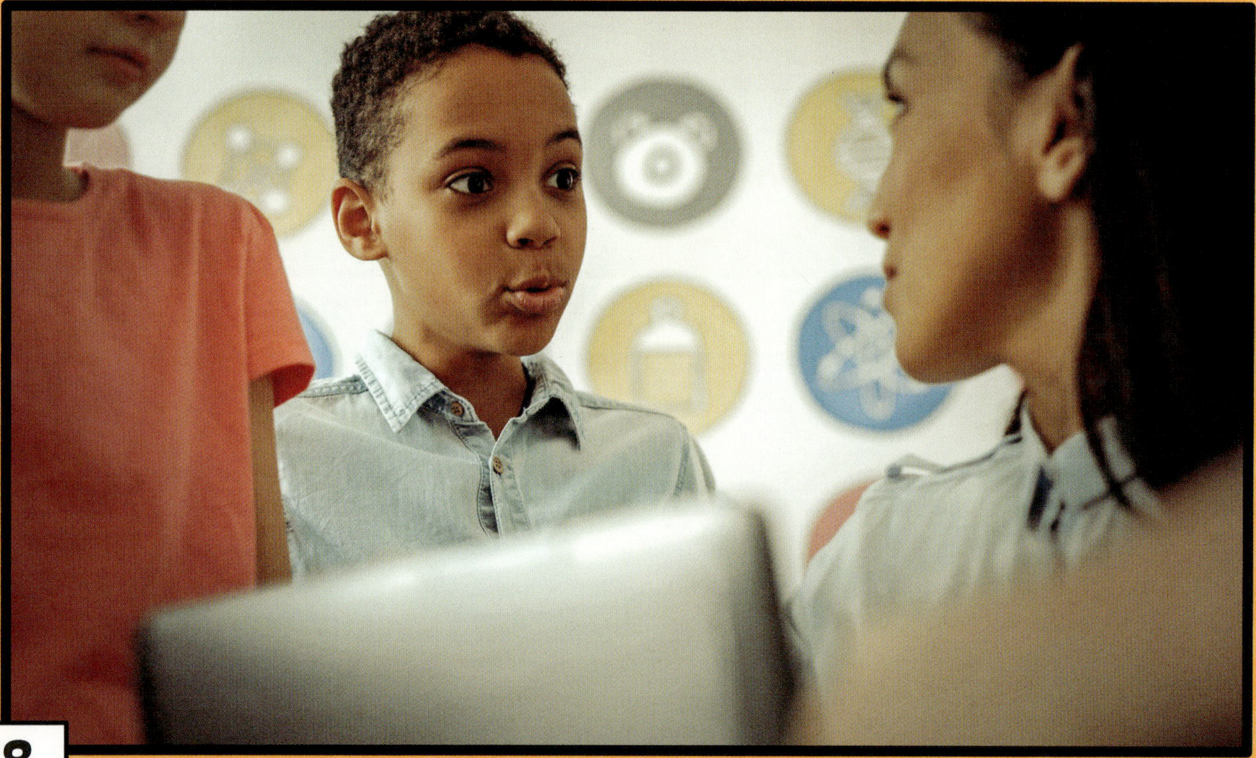

The grown-up will create a safe and calm space for the person with autism. They might turn the lights down or give them headphones to block out sound.

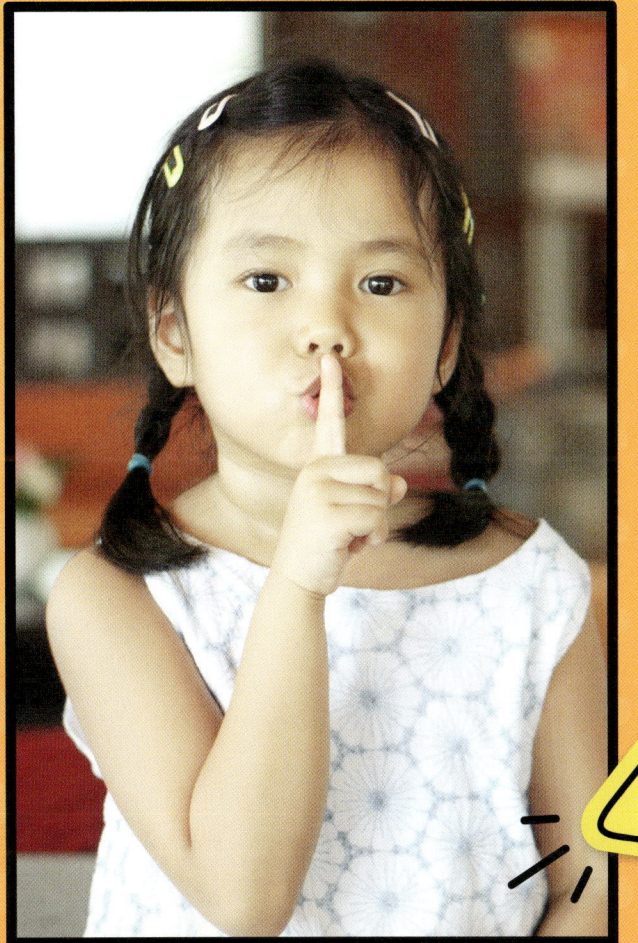

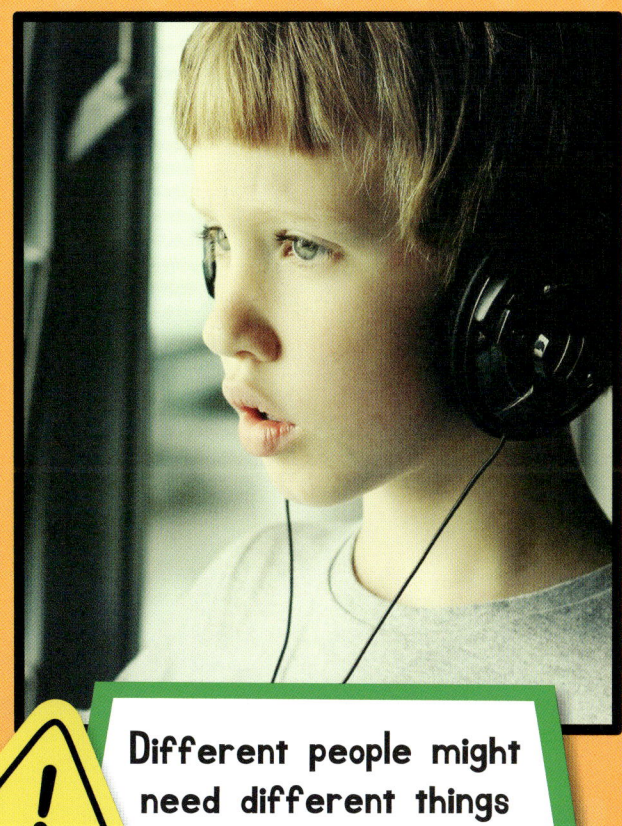

Different people might need different things to calm them.

HOW WE FEEL

A meltdown can be surprising or confusing to see. It is important to stay calm. Be kind when a person with autism has calmed down. It was hard for them, too.

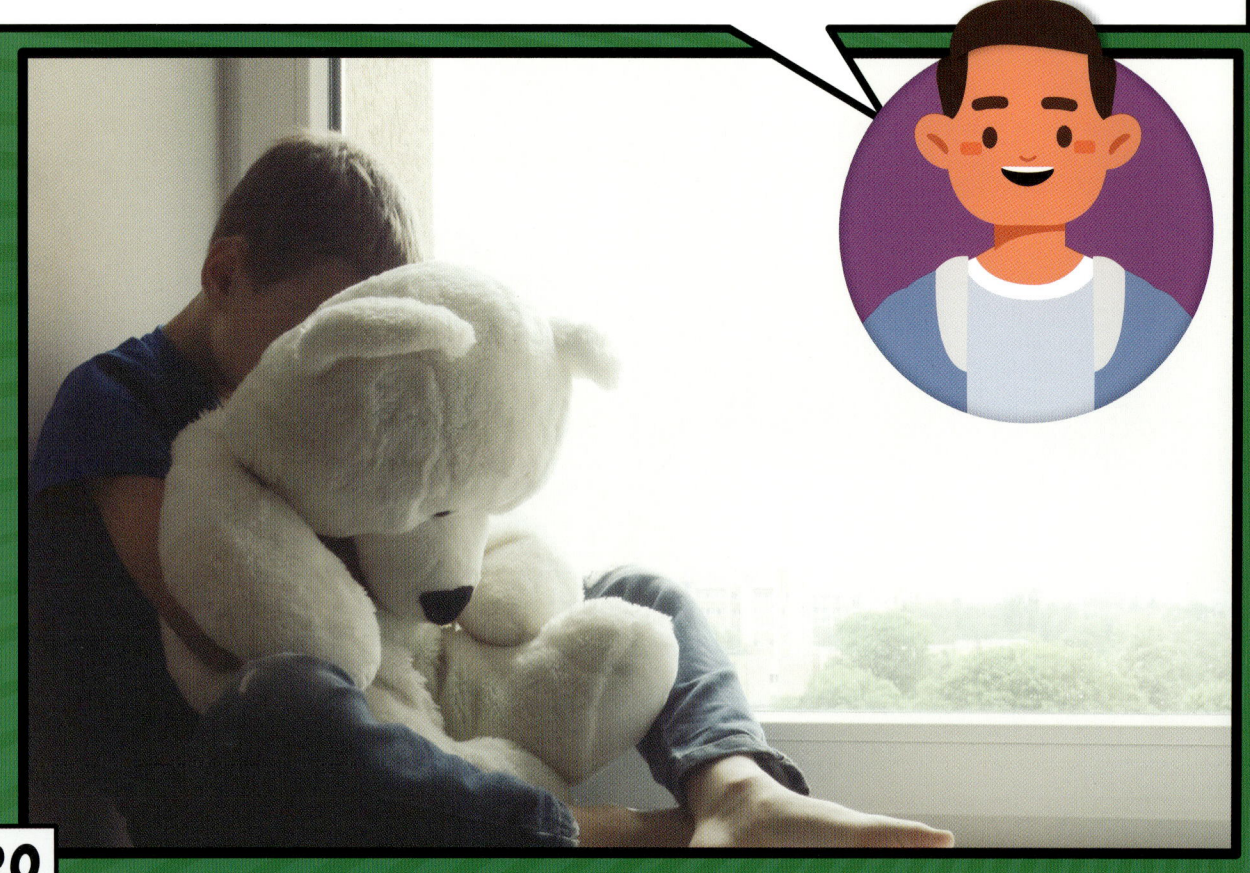

It is never okay to bully someone for being different. Everyone is special in their own way, and everyone needs help with different things.

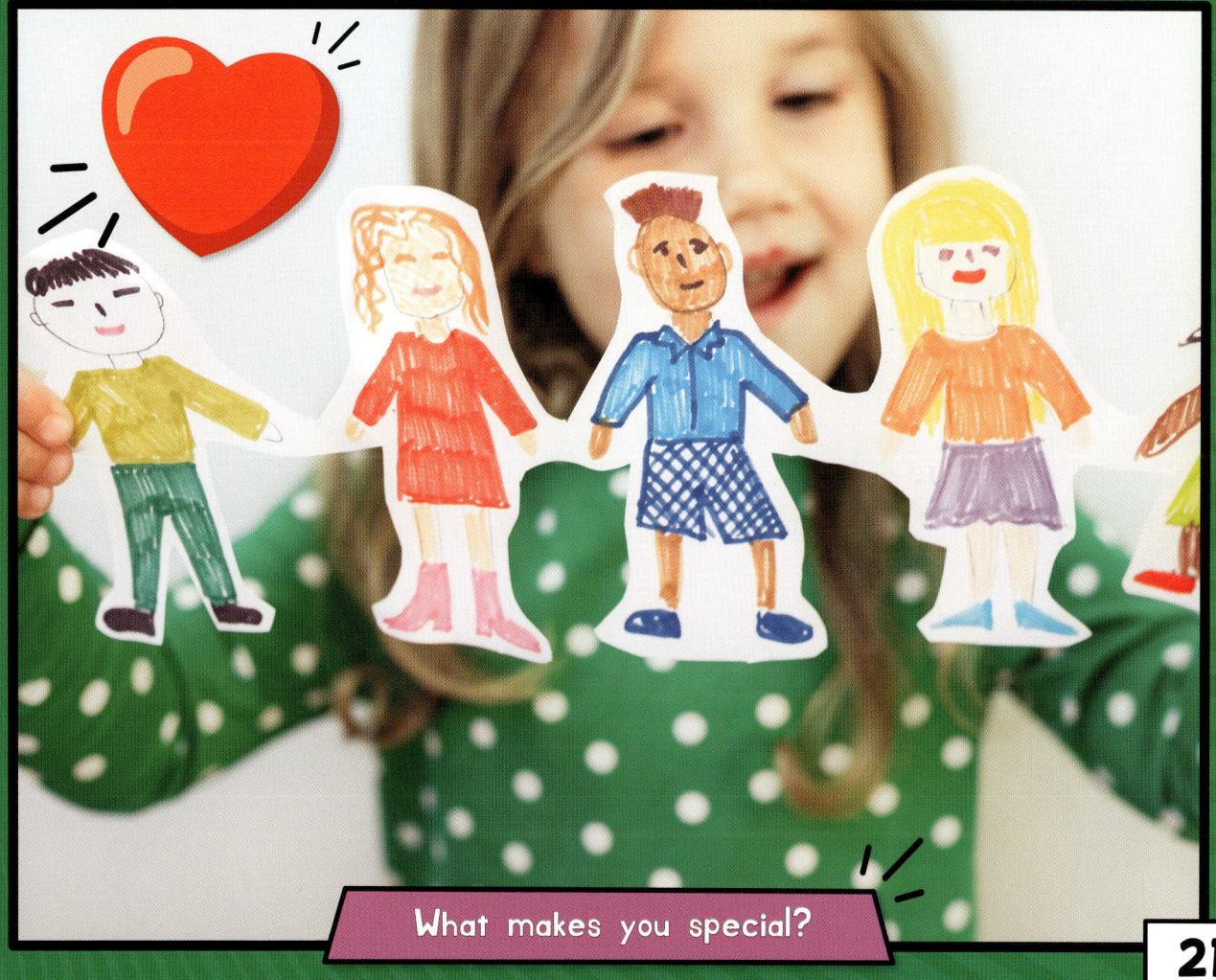

What makes you special?

WHAT NEXT?

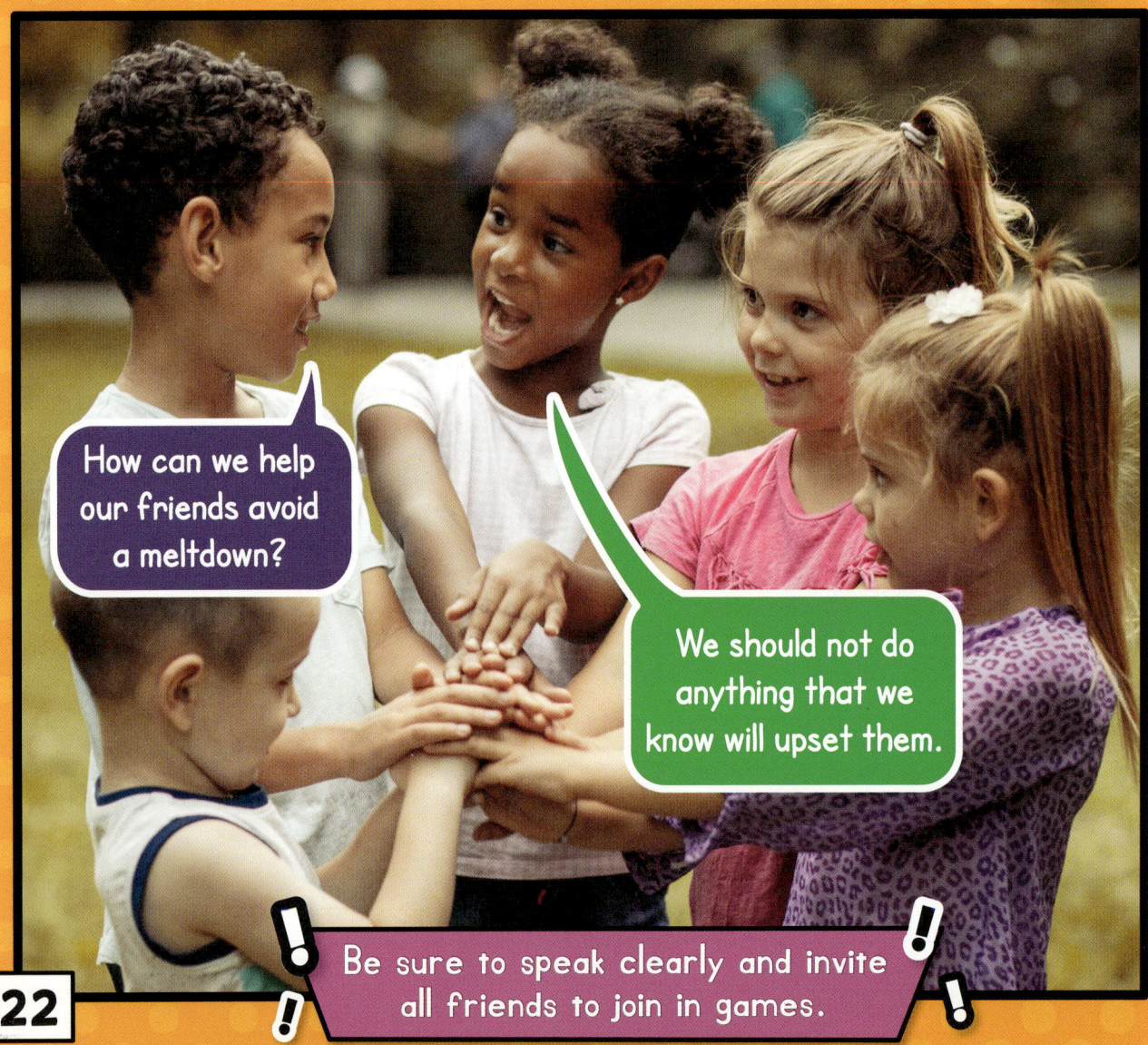

How can we help our friends avoid a meltdown?

We should not do anything that we know will upset them.

Be sure to speak clearly and invite all friends to join in games.

LIVING WITH AUTISM

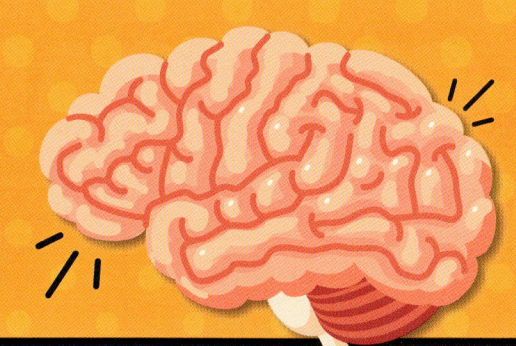

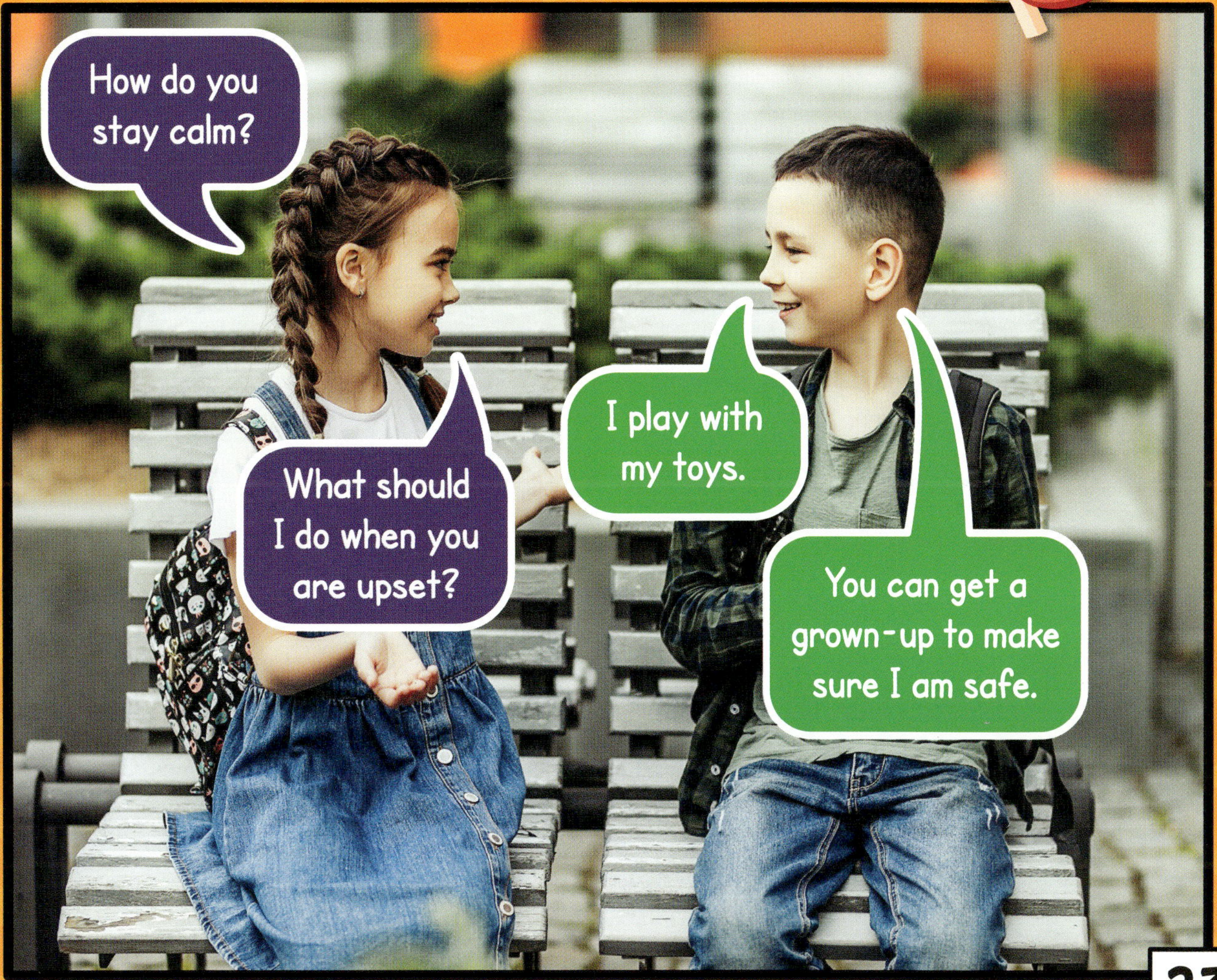

GLOSSARY

anxious worried

communicate to share information with other people

emotions feelings, such as anger, happiness, fear, or sadness

meltdown the big response of someone who is overwhelmed and cannot stay calm

neurotypical thinking about or experiencing the world in the same way as many other people

overwhelmed upset because there is too much happening

routine a regular way of doing something the same way every time

INDEX

brains 6
emergencies 4–5
grown-ups 18–19, 23
lights 13, 19
meltdowns 5, 10–11, 14, 16–18, 20, 22
noises 13
routines 9, 13
smells 13
triggers 12–13